Aivah's Story

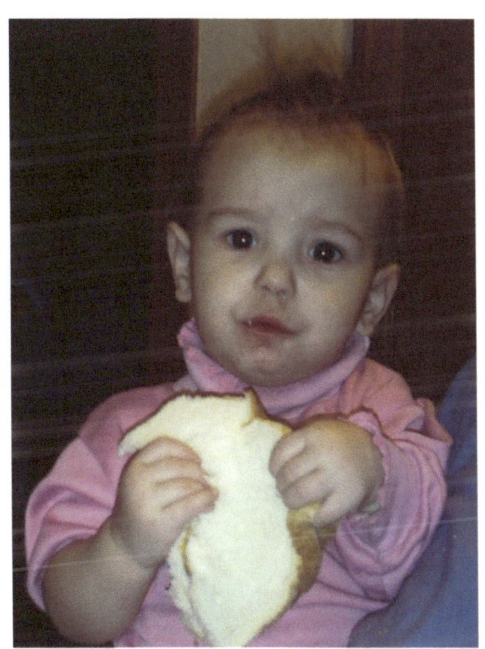

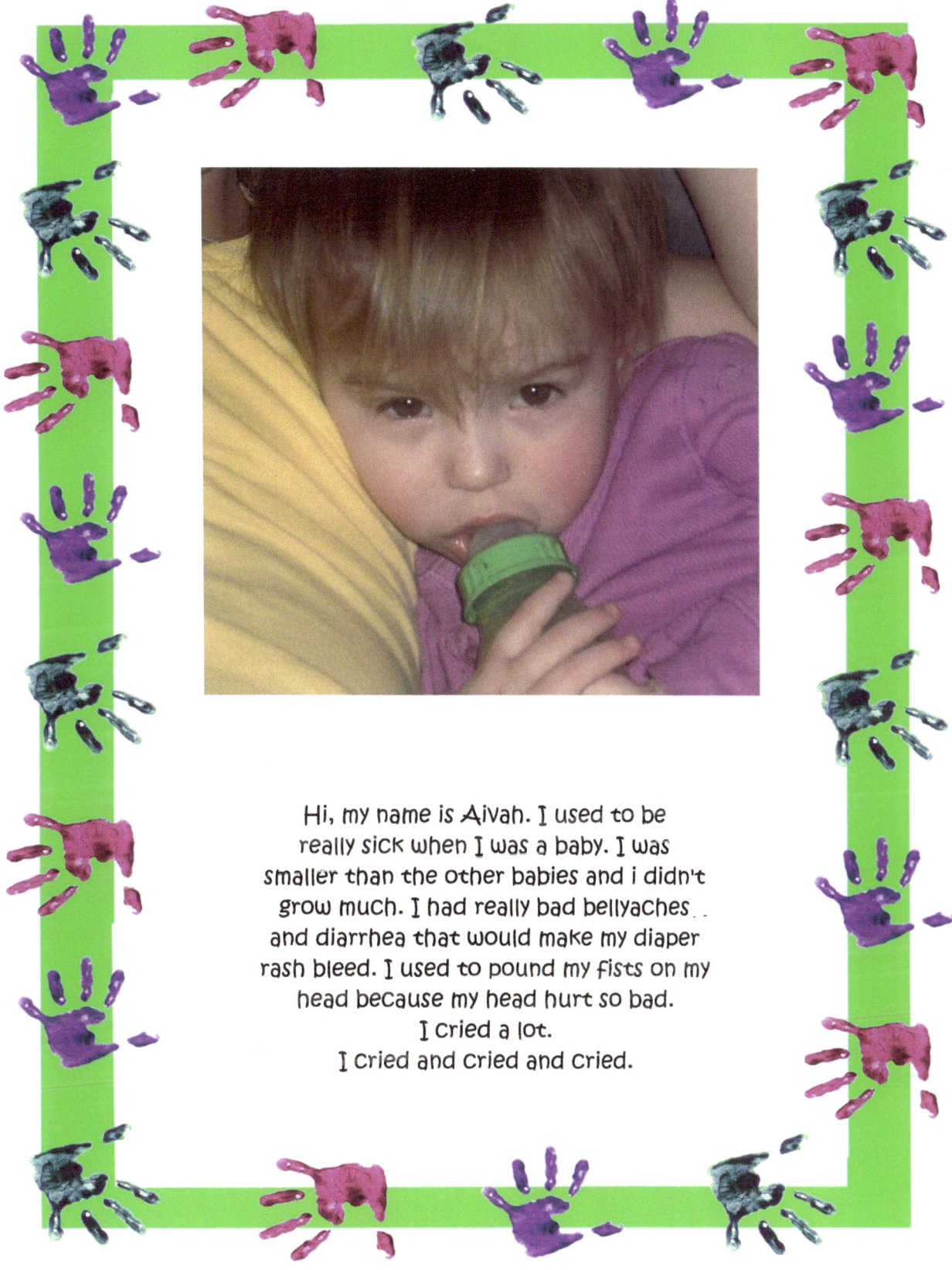

Hi, my name is Aivah. I used to be
really sick when I was a baby. I was
smaller than the other babies and i didn't
grow much. I had really bad bellyaches
and diarrhea that would make my diaper
rash bleed. I used to pound my fists on my
head because my head hurt so bad.
I cried a lot.
I cried and cried and cried.

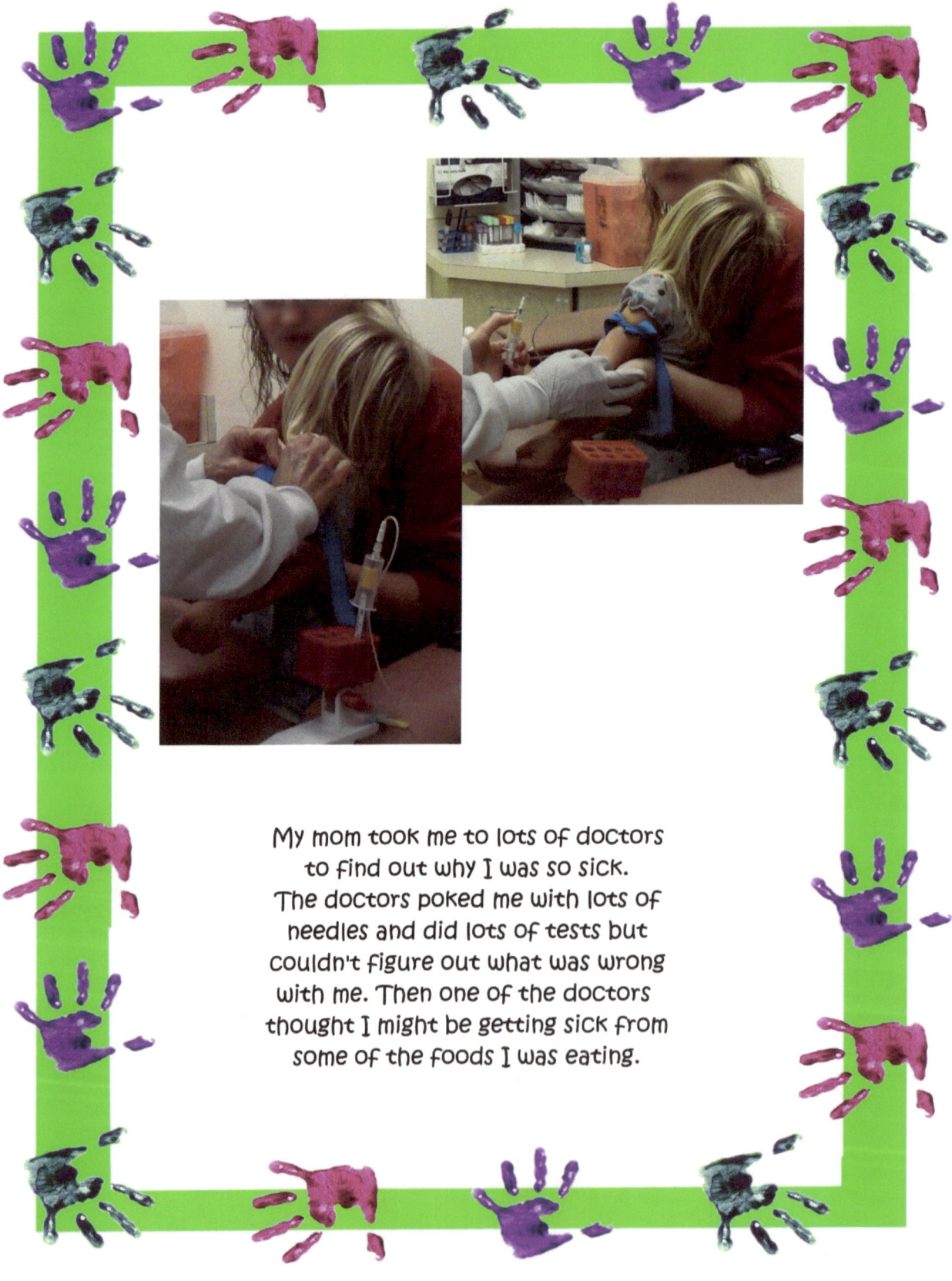

My mom took me to lots of doctors
to find out why I was so sick.
The doctors poked me with lots of
needles and did lots of tests but
couldn't figure out what was wrong
with me. Then one of the doctors
thought I might be getting sick from
some of the foods I was eating.

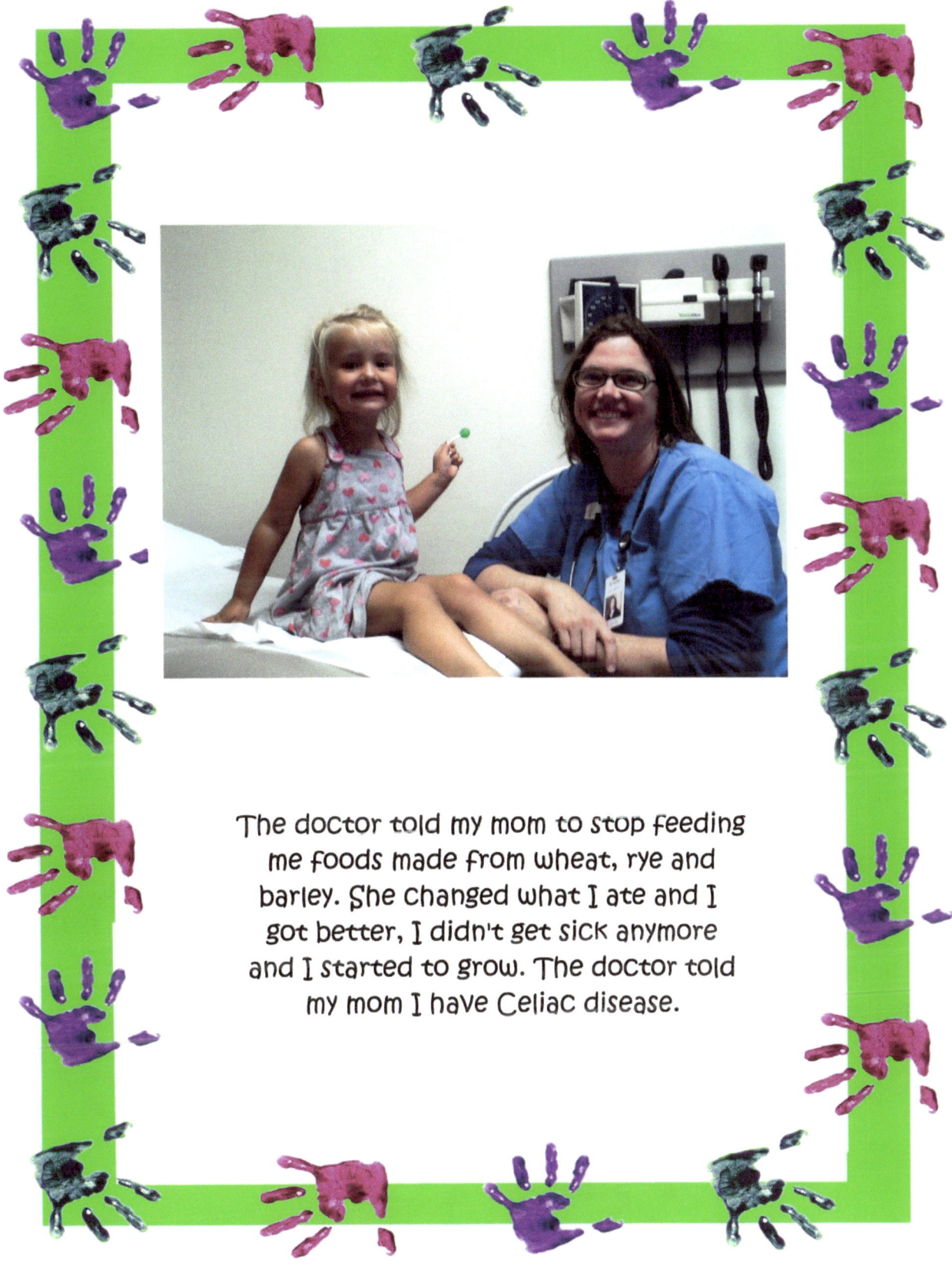

The doctor told my mom to stop feeding
me foods made from wheat, rye and
barley. She changed what I ate and I
got better, I didn't get sick anymore
and I started to grow. The doctor told
my mom I have Celiac disease.

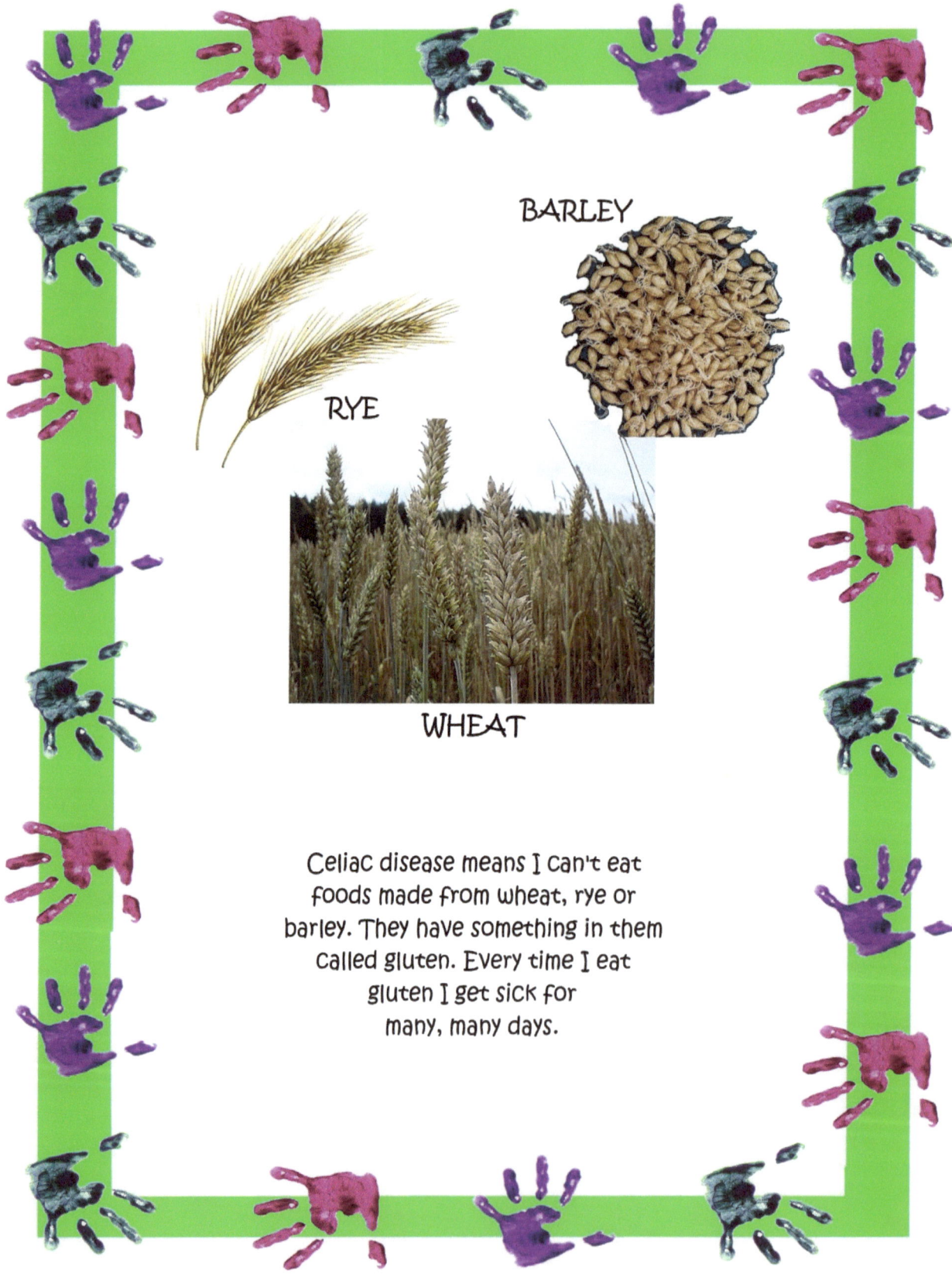

BARLEY

RYE

WHEAT

Celiac disease means I can't eat foods made from wheat, rye or barley. They have something in them called gluten. Every time I eat gluten I get sick for many, many days.

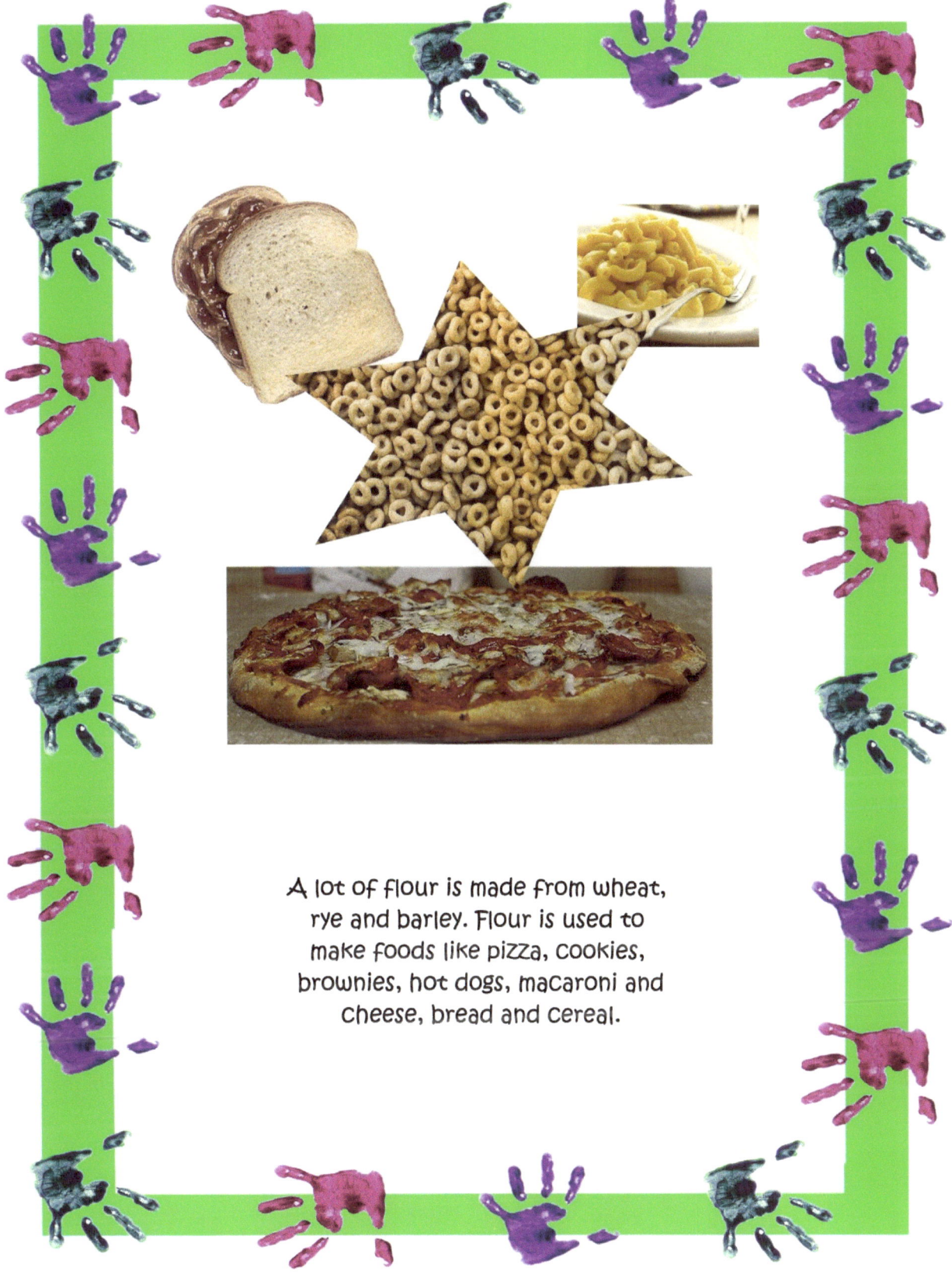

A lot of flour is made from wheat, rye and barley. Flour is used to make foods like pizza, cookies, brownies, hot dogs, macaroni and cheese, bread and cereal.

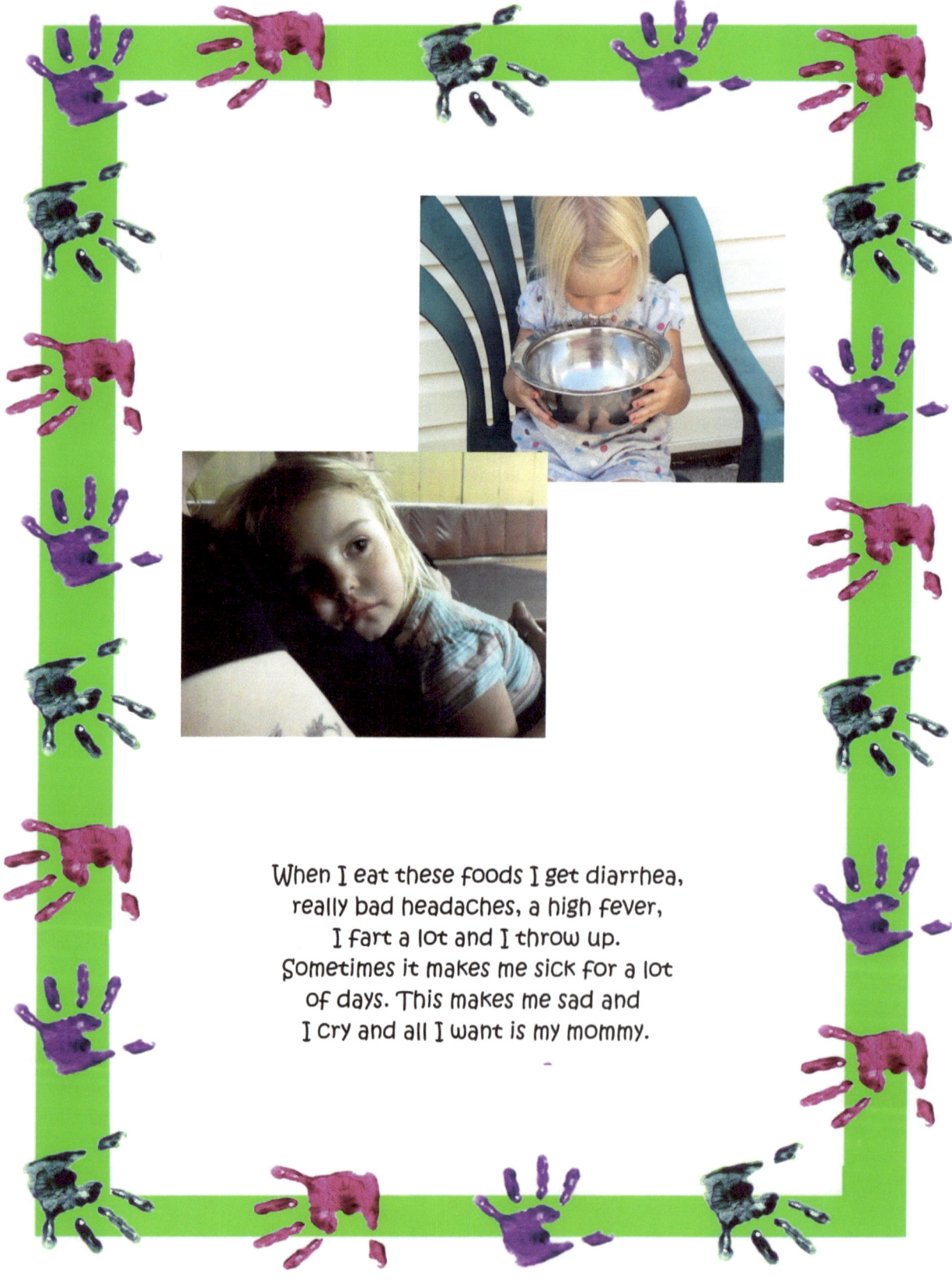

When I eat these foods I get diarrhea,
really bad headaches, a high fever,
I fart a lot and I throw up.
Sometimes it makes me sick for a lot
of days. This makes me sad and
I cry and all I want is my mommy.

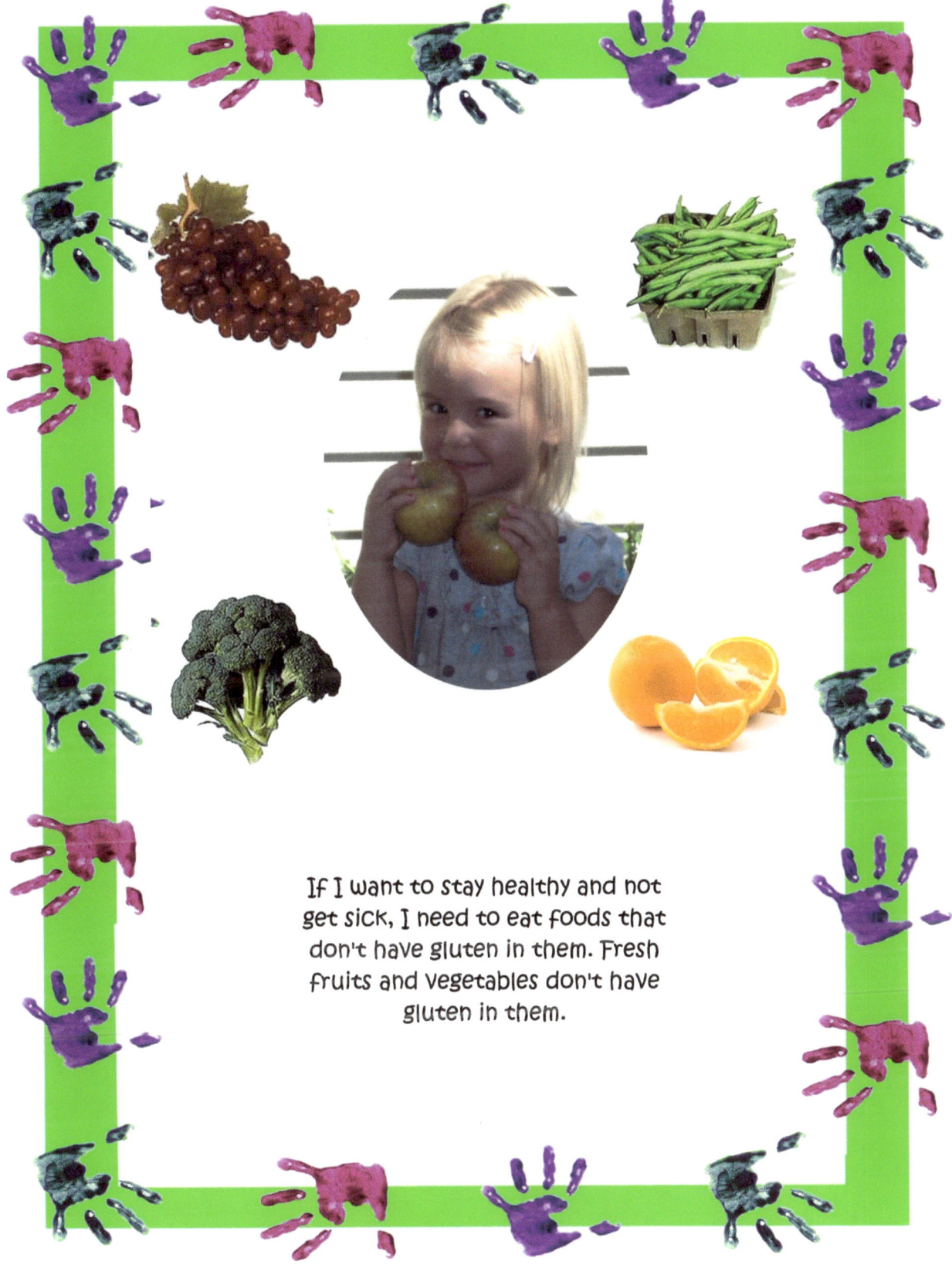

If I want to stay healthy and not get sick, I need to eat foods that don't have gluten in them. Fresh fruits and vegetables don't have gluten in them.

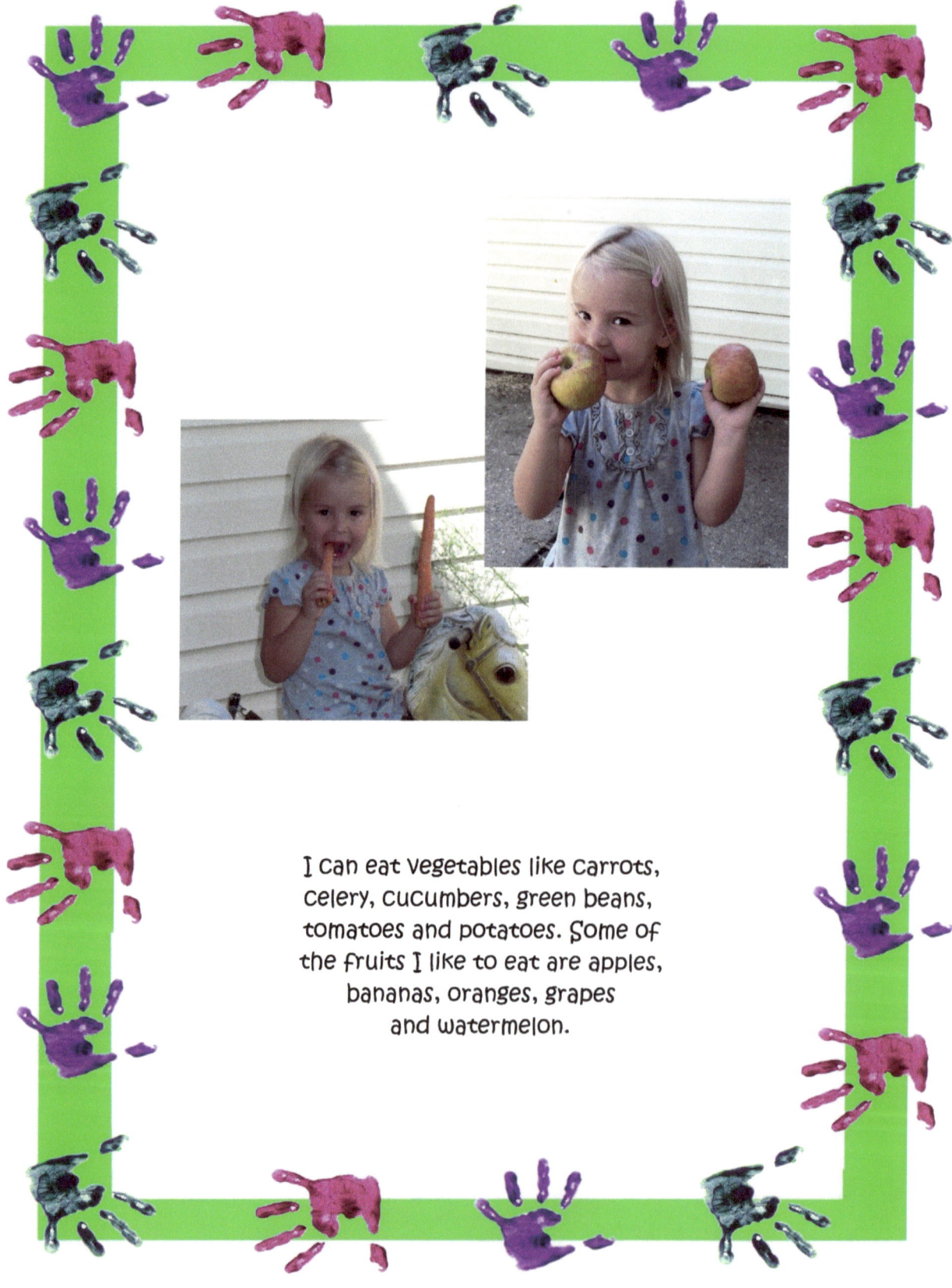

I can eat vegetables like carrots, celery, cucumbers, green beans, tomatoes and potatoes. Some of the fruits I like to eat are apples, bananas, oranges, grapes and watermelon.

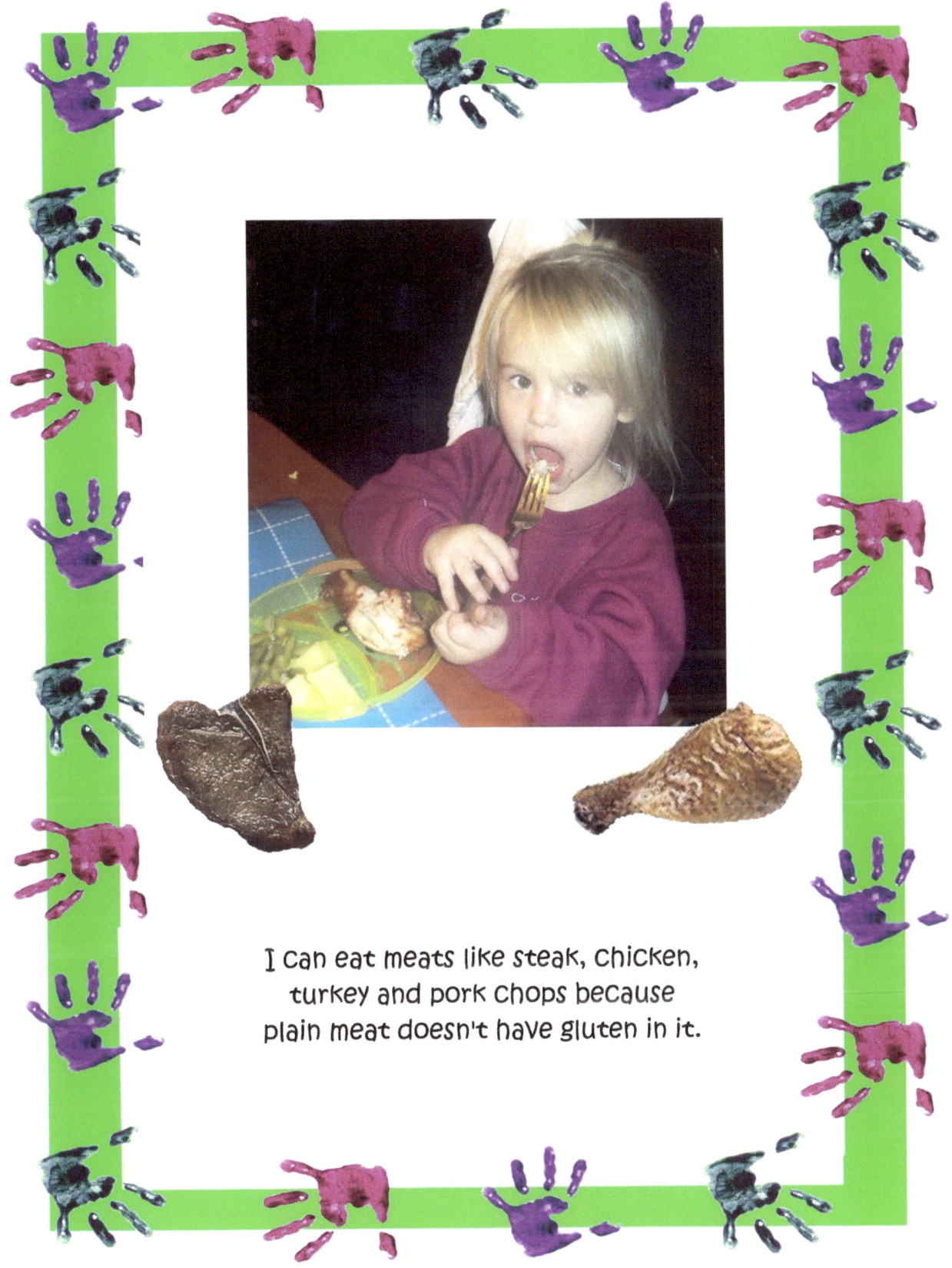

I can eat meats like steak, chicken,
turkey and pork chops because
plain meat doesn't have gluten in it.

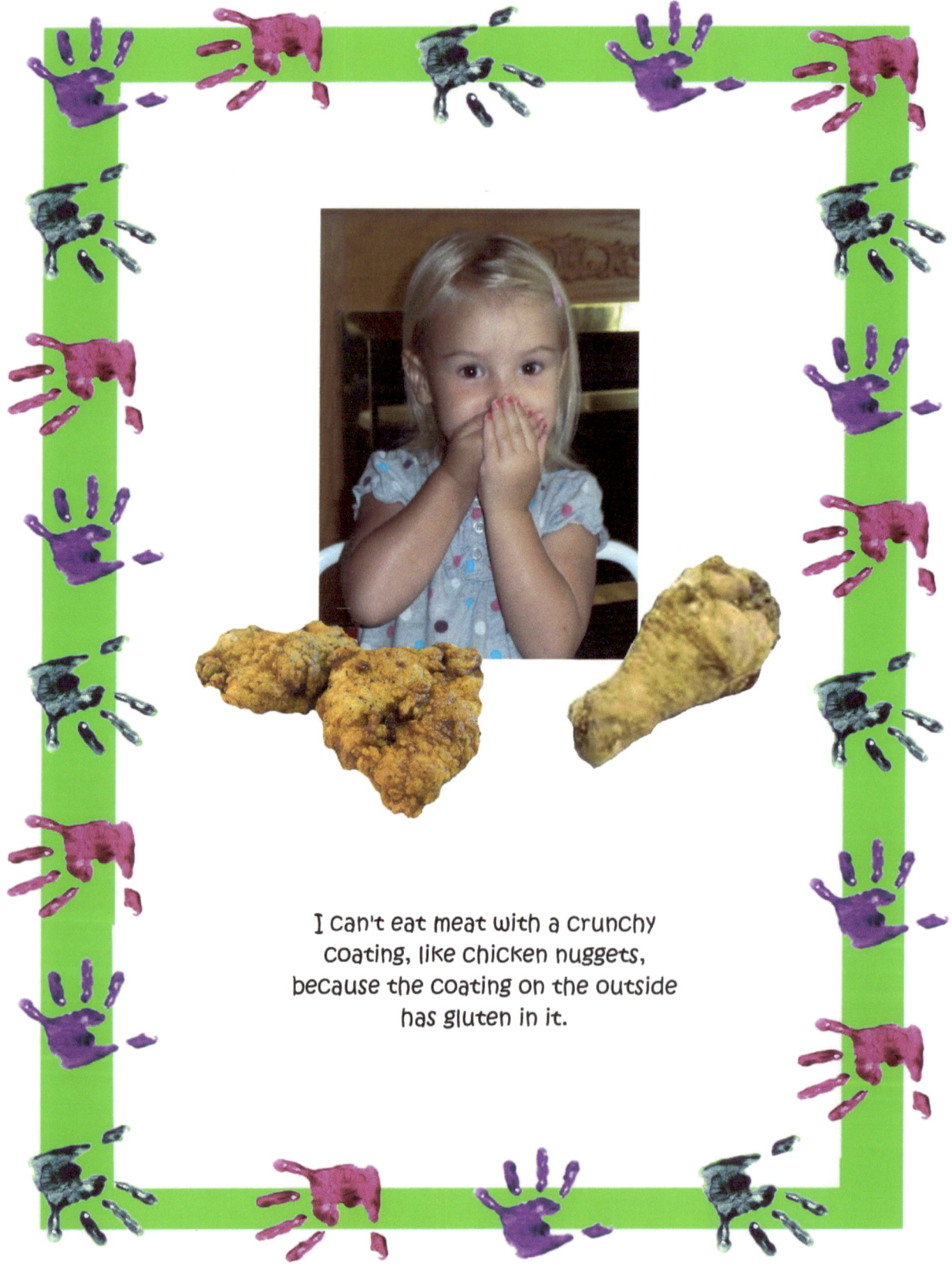

I can't eat meat with a crunchy
coating, like chicken nuggets,
because the coating on the outside
has gluten in it.

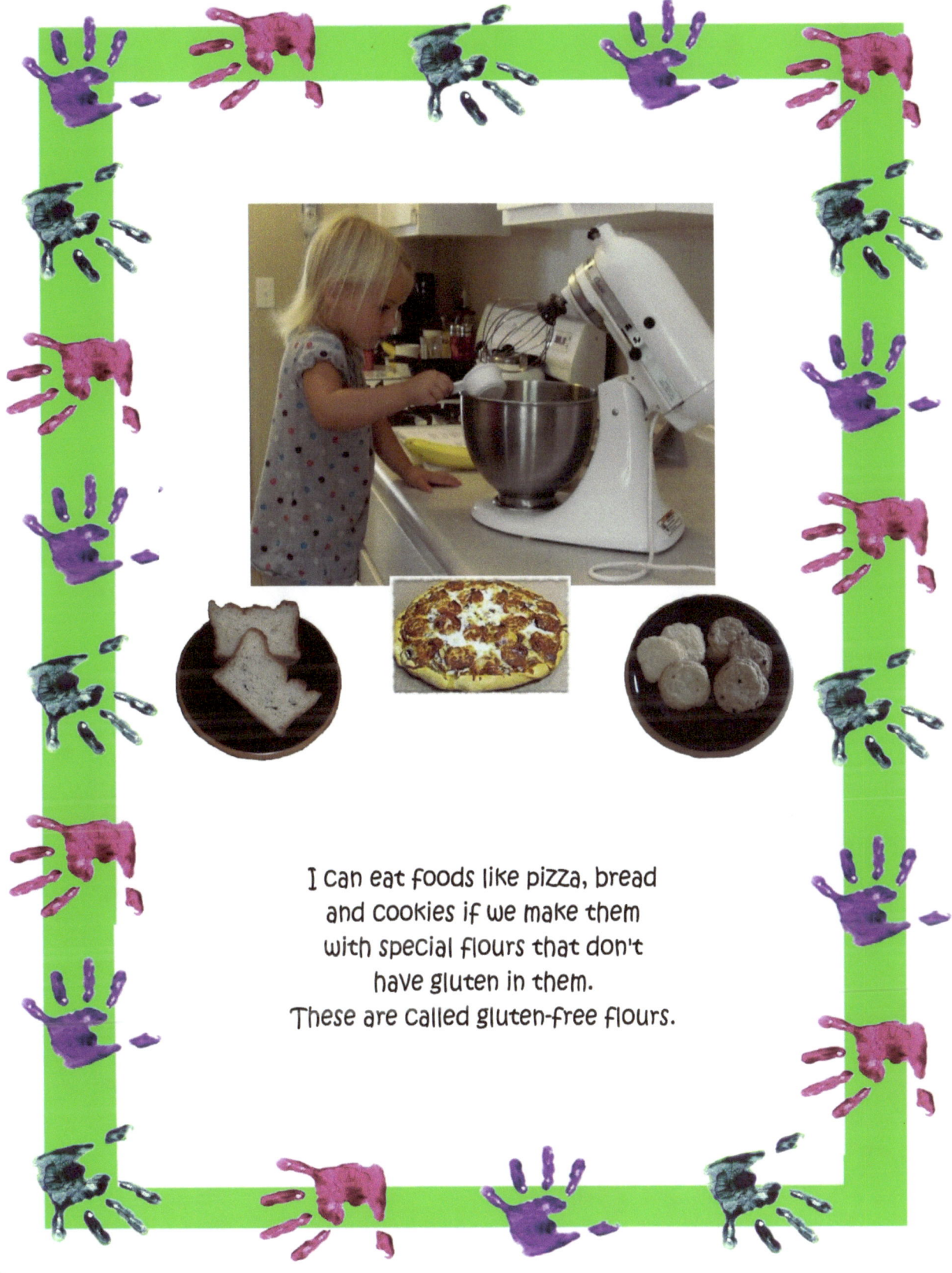

I can eat foods like pizza, bread
and cookies if we make them
with special flours that don't
have gluten in them.
These are called gluten-free flours.

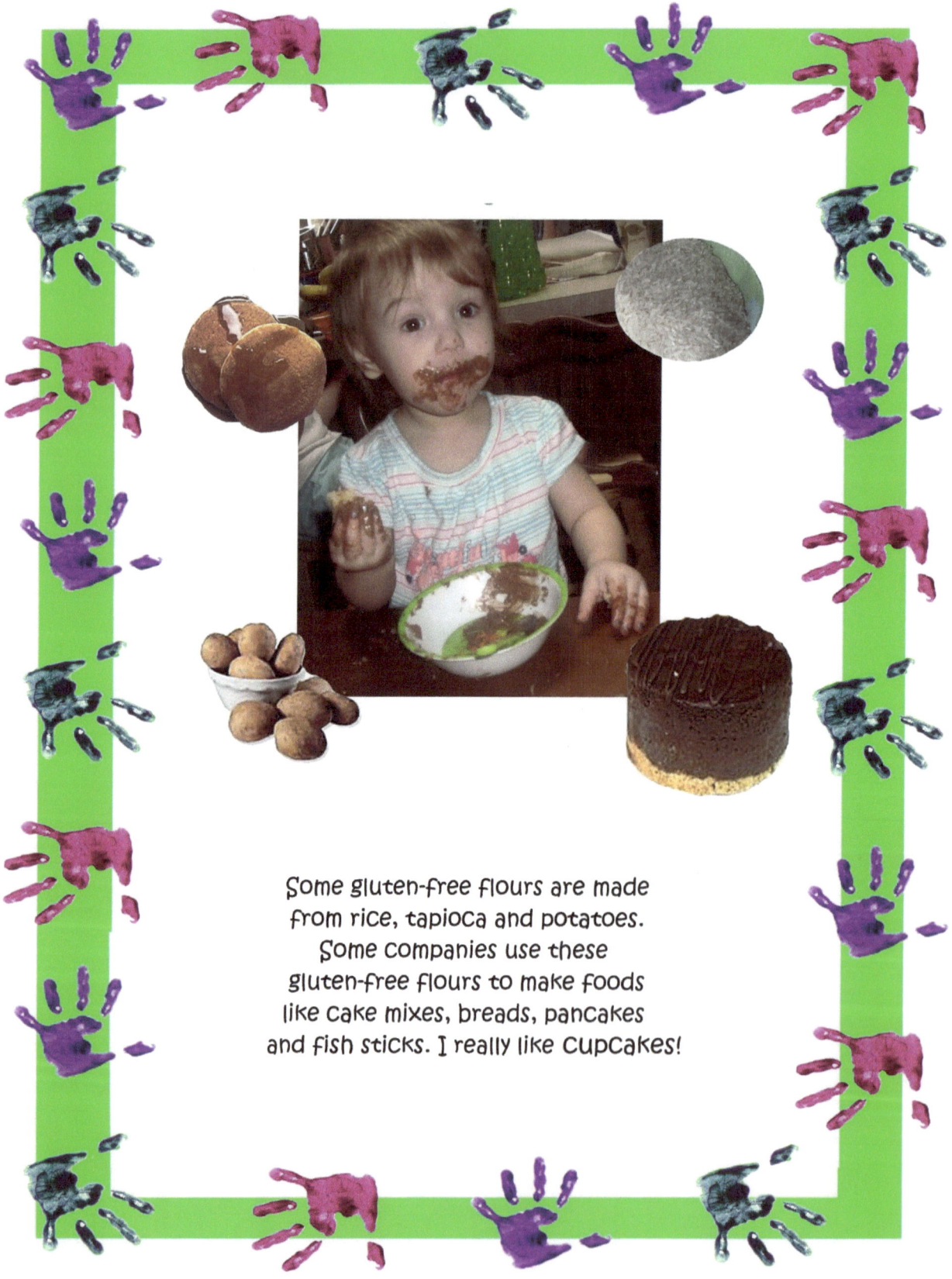

Some gluten-free flours are made
from rice, tapioca and potatoes.
Some companies use these
gluten-free flours to make foods
like cake mixes, breads, pancakes
and fish sticks. I really like cupcakes!

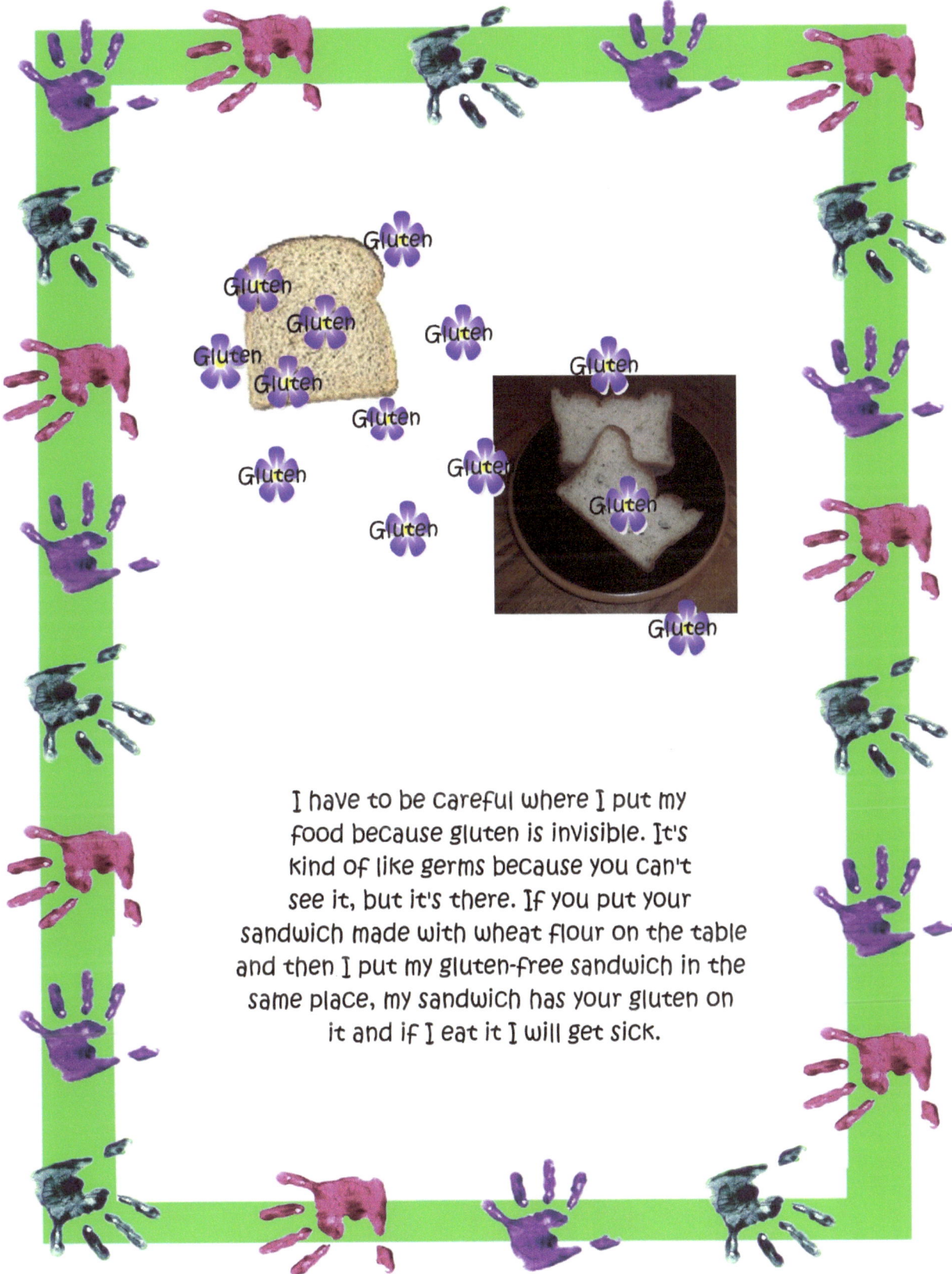

I have to be careful where I put my food because gluten is invisible. It's kind of like germs because you can't see it, but it's there. If you put your sandwich made with wheat flour on the table and then I put my gluten-free sandwich in the same place, my sandwich has your gluten on it and if I eat it I will get sick.

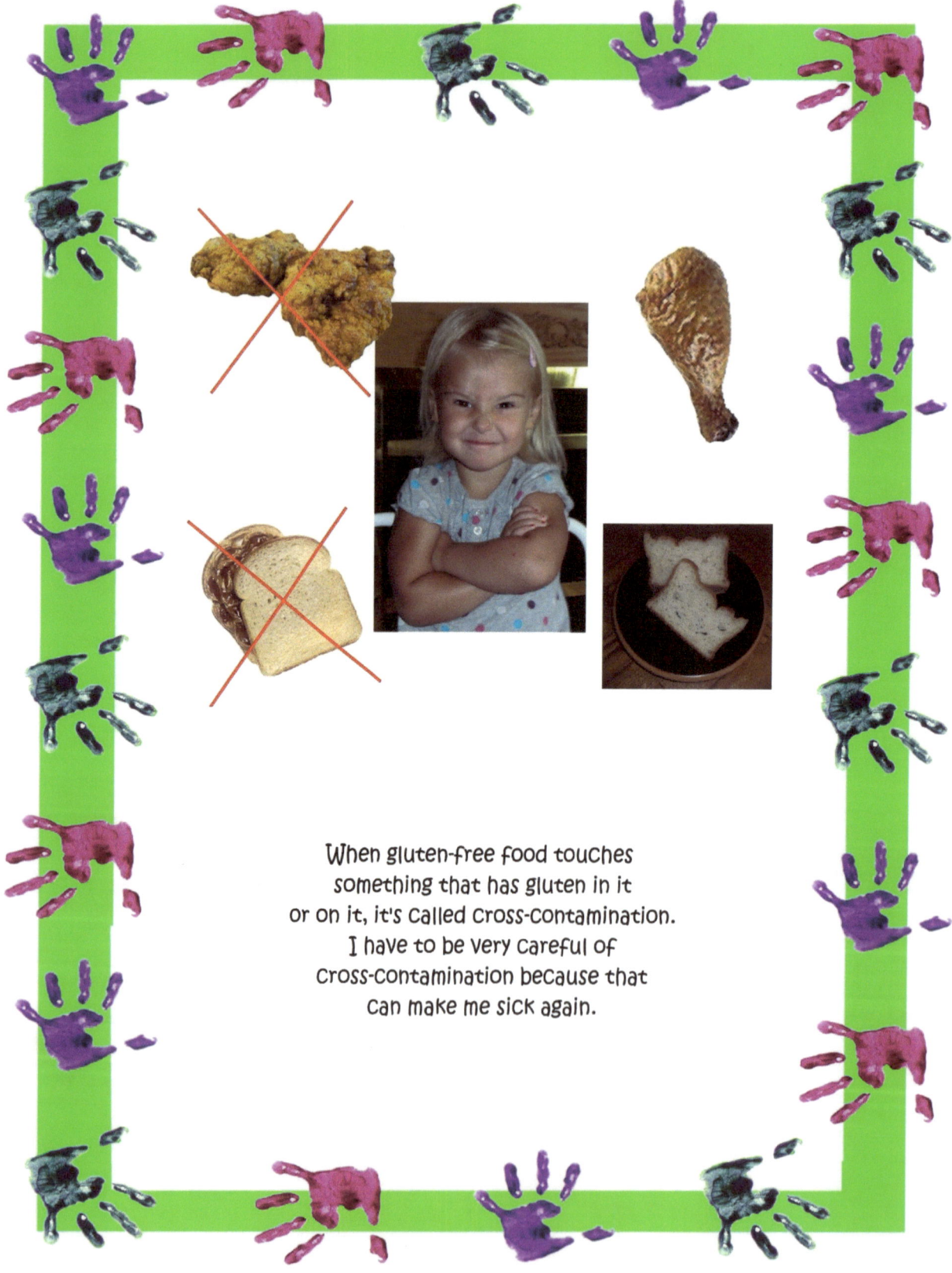

When gluten-free food touches
something that has gluten in it
or on it, it's called cross-contamination.
I have to be very careful of
cross-contamination because that
can make me sick again.

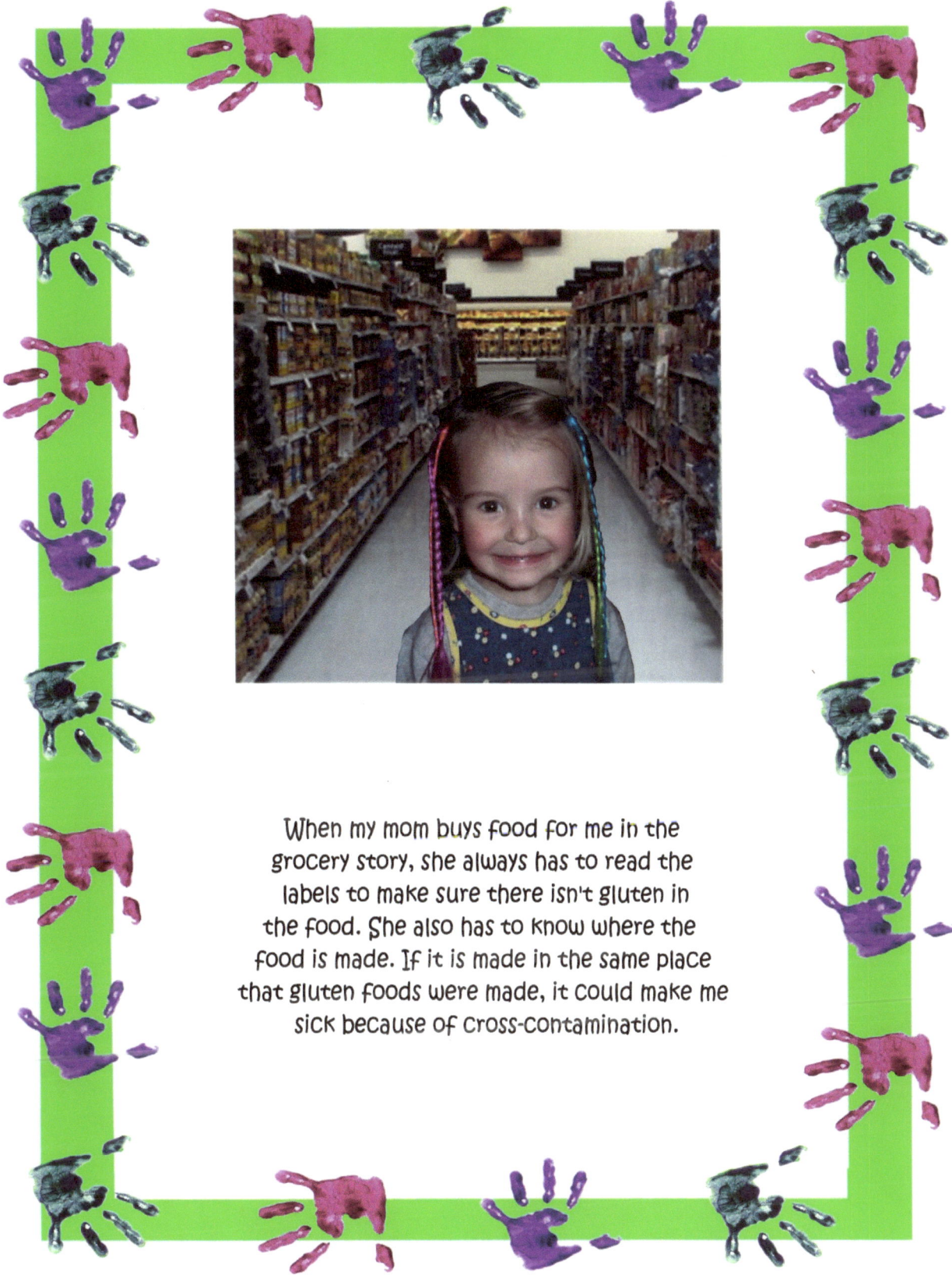

When my mom buys food for me in the grocery story, she always has to read the labels to make sure there isn't gluten in the food. She also has to know where the food is made. If it is made in the same place that gluten foods were made, it could make me sick because of cross-contamination.

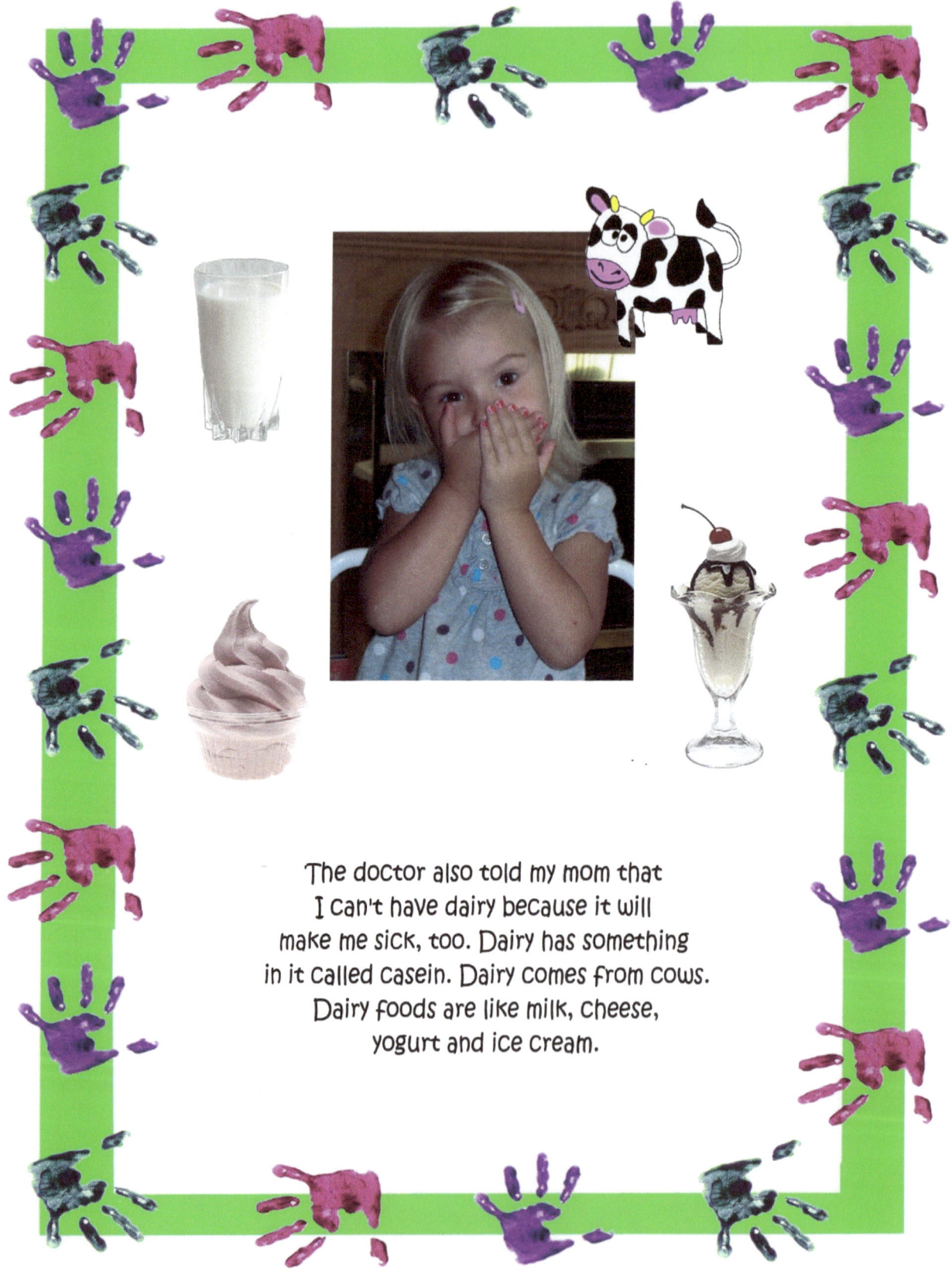

The doctor also told my mom that
I can't have dairy because it will
make me sick, too. Dairy has something
in it called casein. Dairy comes from cows.
Dairy foods are like milk, cheese,
yogurt and ice cream.

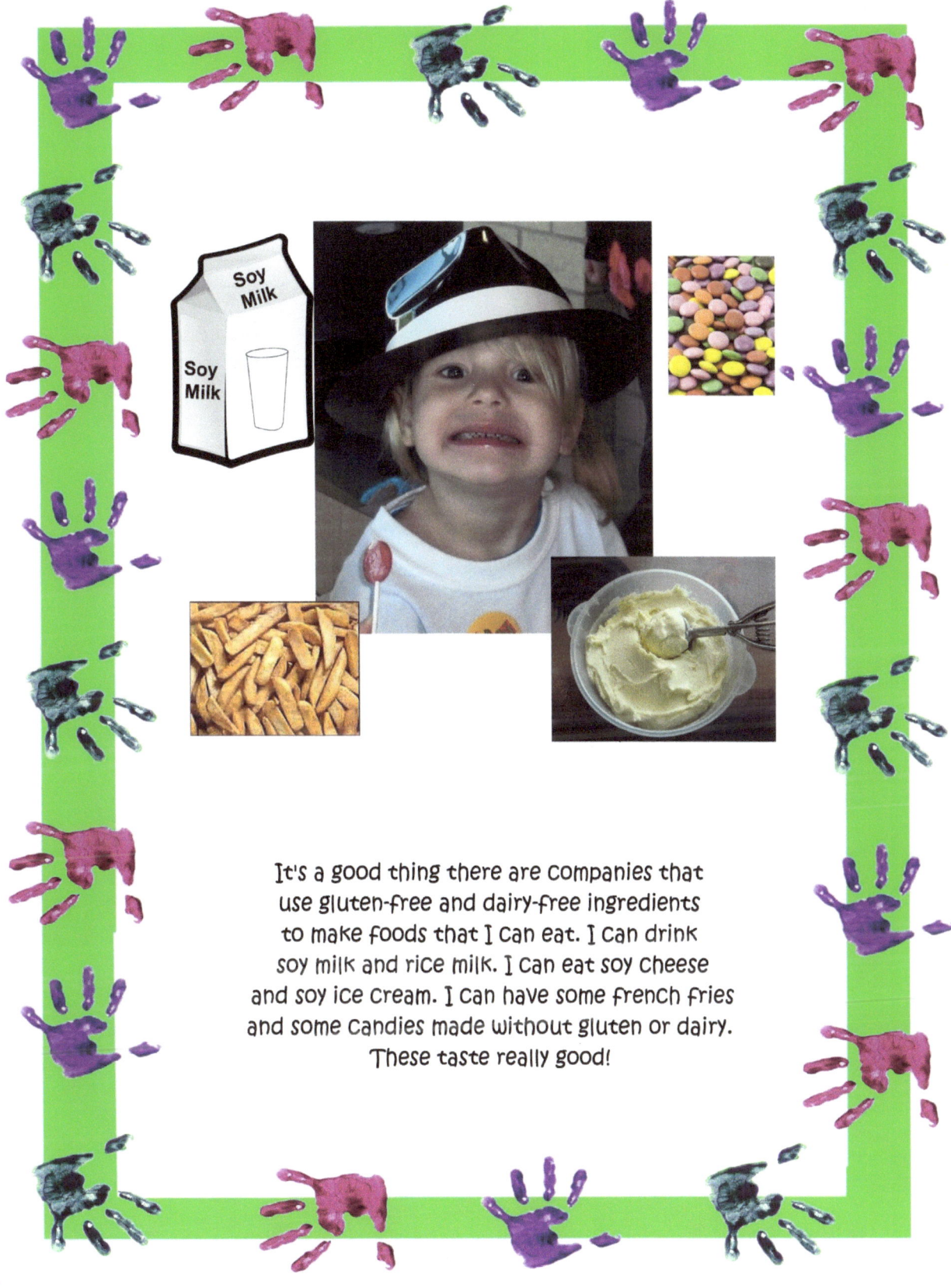

It's a good thing there are companies that use gluten-free and dairy-free ingredients to make foods that I can eat. I can drink soy milk and rice milk. I can eat soy cheese and soy ice cream. I can have some french fries and some candies made without gluten or dairy. These taste really good!

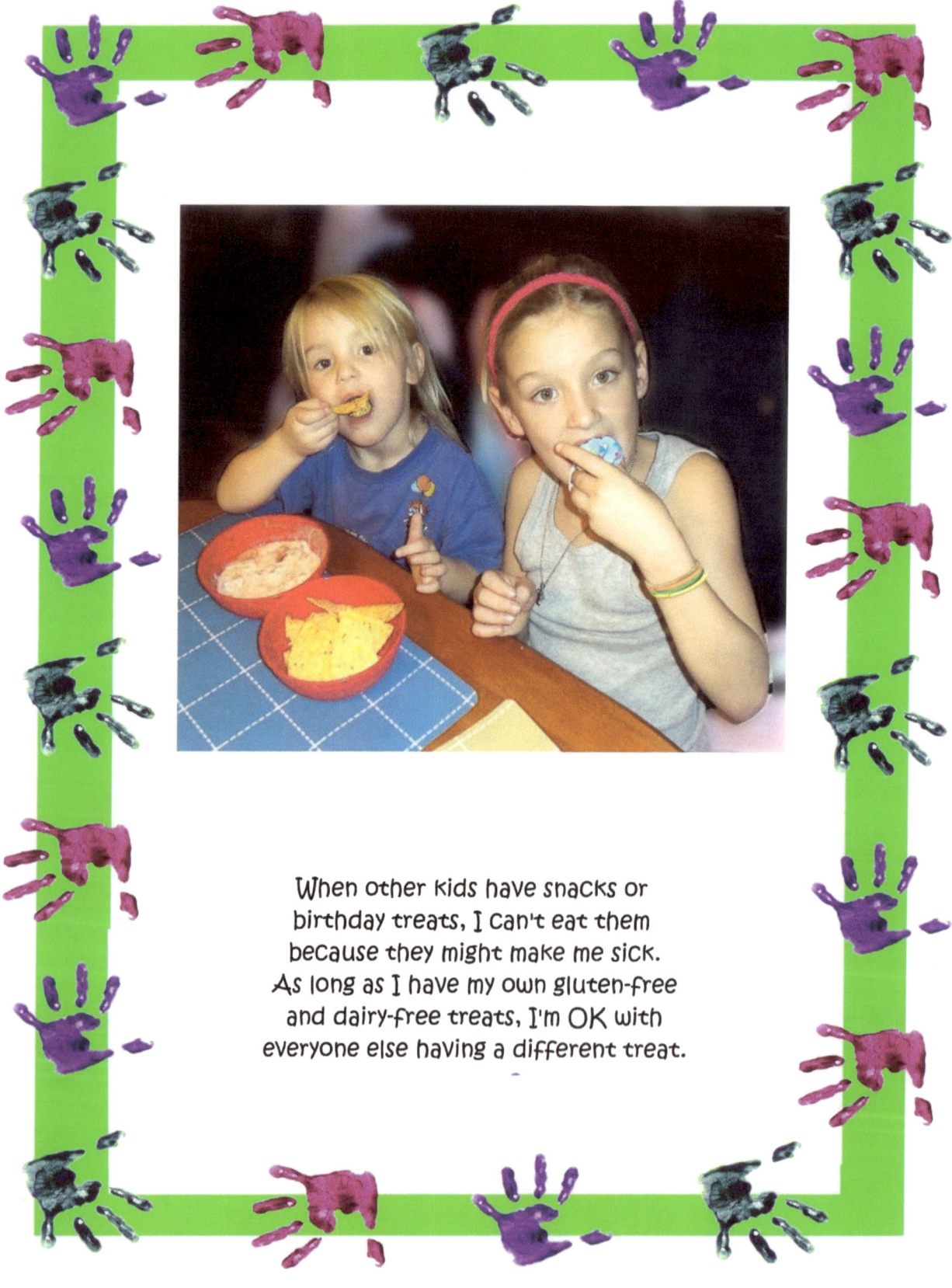

When other kids have snacks or
birthday treats, I can't eat them
because they might make me sick.
As long as I have my own gluten-free
and dairy-free treats, I'm OK with
everyone else having a different treat.

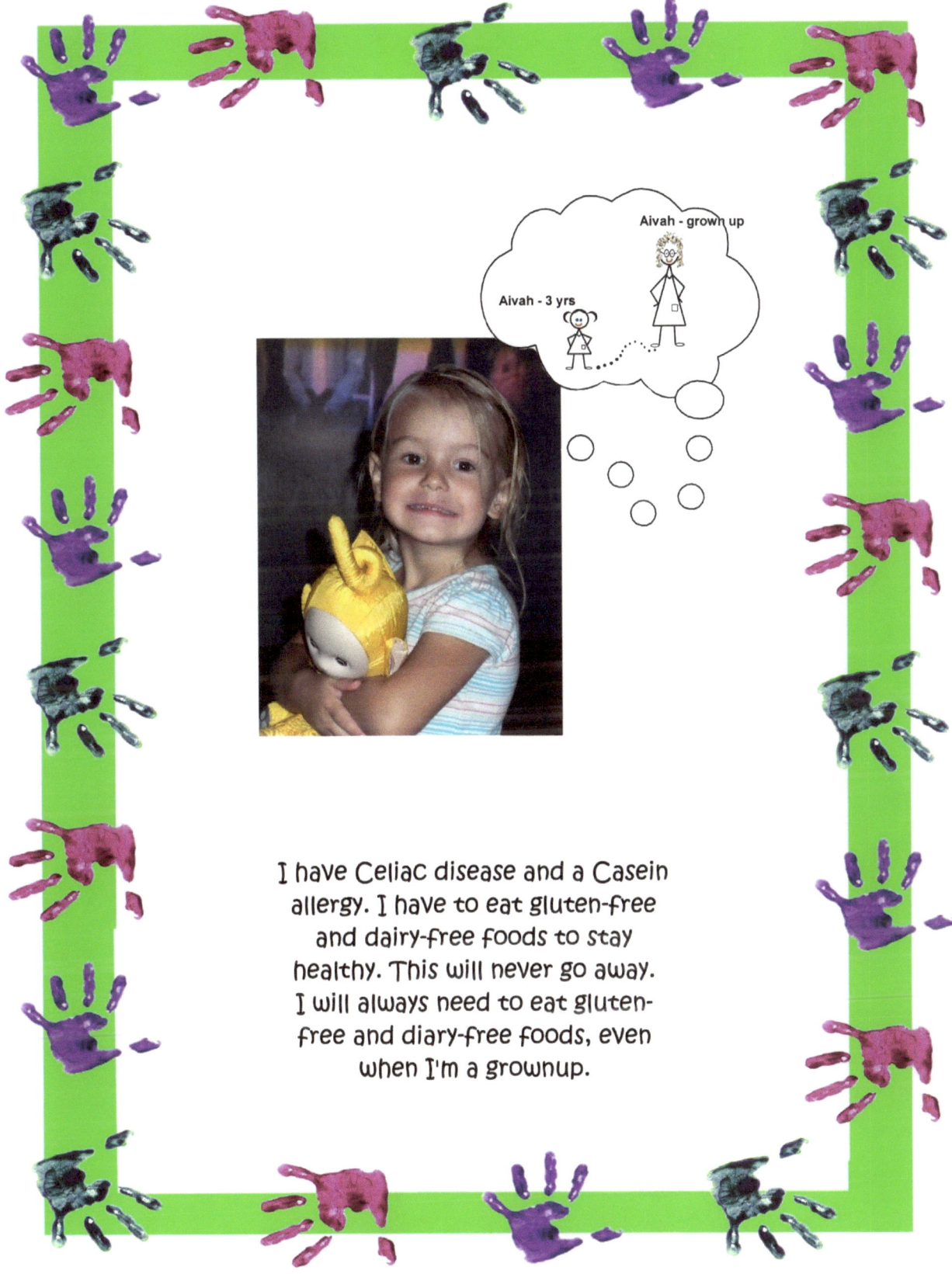

I have Celiac disease and a Casein allergy. I have to eat gluten-free and dairy-free foods to stay healthy. This will never go away. I will always need to eat gluten-free and diary-free foods, even when I'm a grownup.

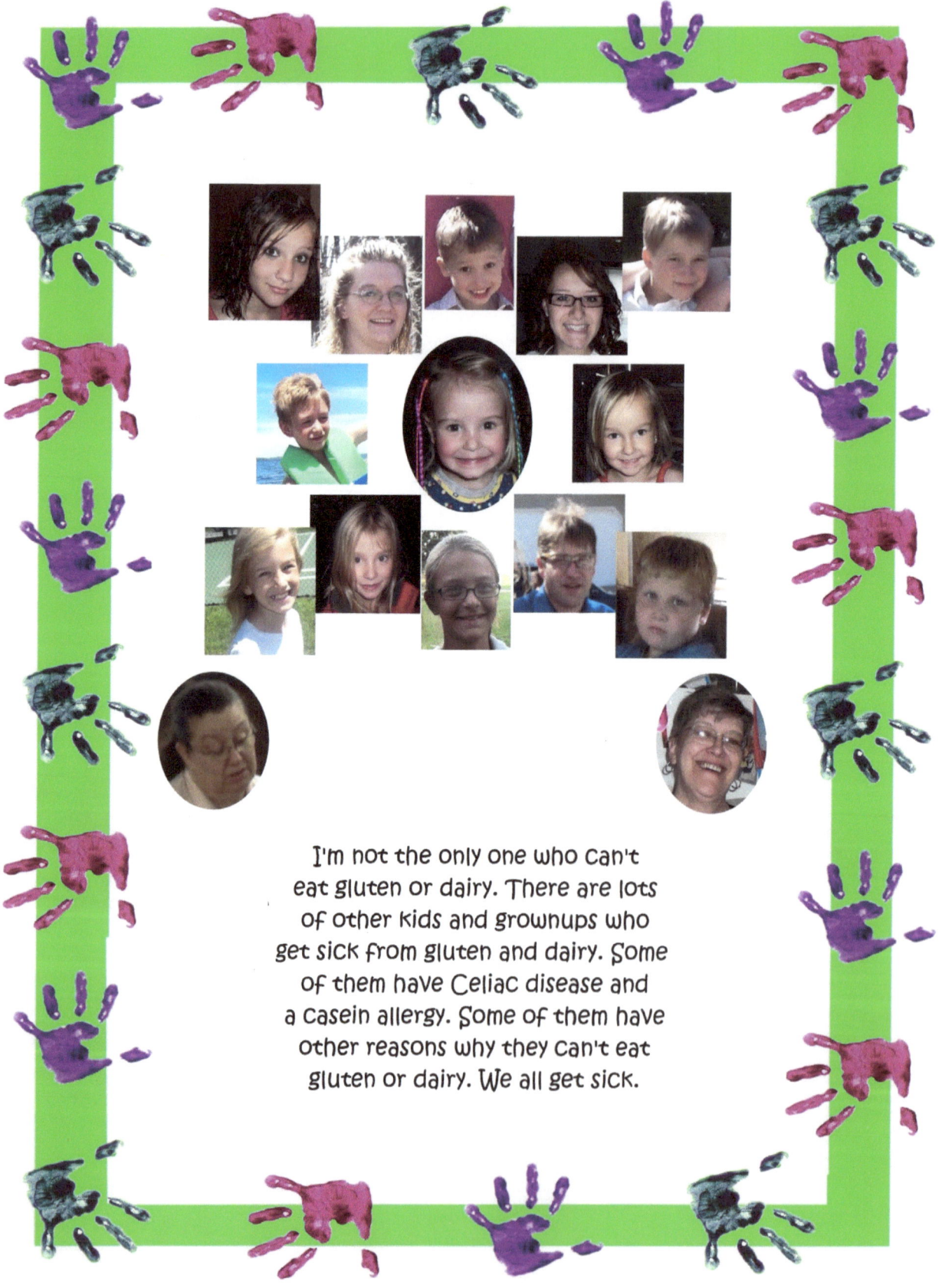

I'm not the only one who can't
eat gluten or dairy. There are lots
of other kids and grownups who
get sick from gluten and dairy. Some
of them have Celiac disease and
a casein allergy. Some of them have
other reasons why they can't eat
gluten or dairy. We all get sick.

RECIPES

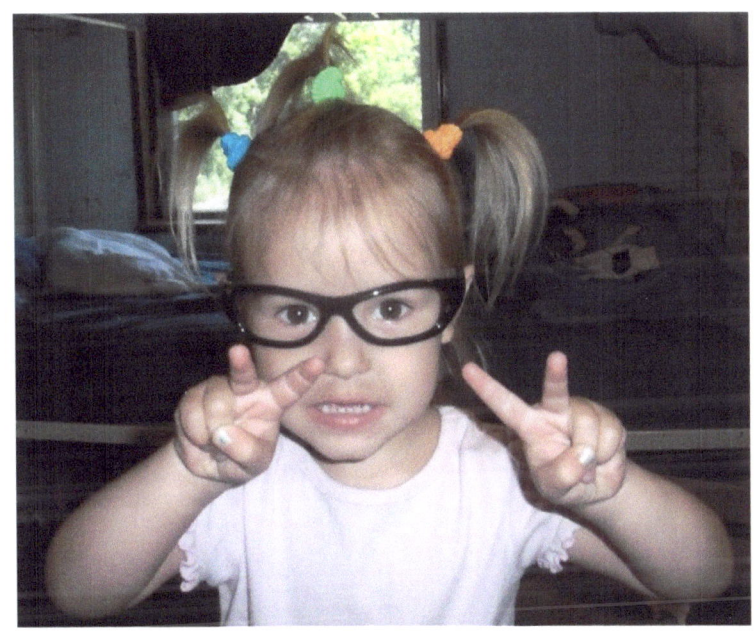

There are many cookbooks available that have gluten-free, dairy- free or gluten-free AND dairy-free recipes.

("Don't Feed Me – Gluten-free, Dairy-free Cooking" is excellent for children and adults who are starting their journey on the gluten-free, dairy-free lifestyle.)

Aivah has her favorite recipes for foods she really likes to eat. She shared her story with you and she would like to share her recipes with you.

We hope they will be your favorites, too.

HAPPY SNACKS

Makes 4 smiles

1 apple
Homemade marshmallows, cut into ¼" squares
GF peanut butter

Cut apple into quarters. Cut out core from each piece. Slice each quarter
in half, lengthwise (you will have 8 pieces.)

Spread peanut butter on one side of each apple slice. Top four of the
slices with marshmallow pieces. (Line them up like teeth.)

Put apple slice without "teeth" on top of the marshmallows, forming a "smile".

CHOCOLATE MAYONNAISE CUPCAKES

Makes about 20 cupcakes

½ C corn or potato starch	1 pkg unflavored gelatin
½ C brown rice flour	1 ½ tsp xanthan gum
1 C tapioca flour	1-2/3 C granulated sugar
2/3 C unsweetened cocoa	1 tsp GF baking powder
1 ½ tsp GF baking soda 3 eggs	
1 C GF mayonnaise	1 1/3 C water

Preheat oven to 350 degrees. Place cupcake papers into cupcake pan (or grease & sugar cups in cupcake pan).
In large bowl combine eggs and sugar. Mix on high for 2 – 3 minutes until light and fluffy and pale yellow. Reduce to low and blend in mayonnaise.

Add 1/3 C water and the soy and rice flours. Mix until well blended. Add another 1/3 C water and tapioca flour, mixing until well blended. Mix in remaining 2/3 C water. Add potato starch flour, gelatin, baking soda, baking powder and cocoa. Mix until well blended. Mix in gelatin and xanthan gum. Mixture will thicken once the xanthan gum is added.

Fill cupcake papers 2/3 full. Bake for 20 minutes or until top springs back when pressed gently.

CREAM PUFFS

Makes 12 puffs

1 C water
½ C GFDF margarine
1/3 C potato starch flour
1/3 C white rice flour
1/3 C tapioca flour
½ tsp salt
1 Tbl granulated sugar
4 eggs

Preheat oven to 450 degrees. Grease cookie sheet.

Combine water and margarine in medium saucepan. Bring to a rapid boil. In medium bowl, mix flours, salt and sugar. Add flour mixture all at one time to boiling water. Turn off heat. Stir vigorously until mixture forms a ball that leaves side of pan. Set pan aside and cool slightly.

Add eggs, one at a time, beating well with wooden spoon after each egg.

Drop 12 spoonsful onto prepared cookie sheet. Bake for 20 minutes, then reduce heat to 350 degrees and bake for 15 – 20 minutes longer. Remove from oven and prick with knife to let steam escape.

Serve cold filled with Dairy-Free Chocolate Pudding (recipe follows) or fill with dairy-free whipped topping.

GLUTEN-FREE, CASEIN-FREE CHOCOLATE PUDDING

Makes 2 ½ cups

3 Tbl cornstarch
2 Tbl water
1 ½ C soy milk (or rice or almond milk)
¼ C granulated sugar
¼ C unsweetened cocoa

In large saucepan whisk ingredients together. Heat over medium heat, stirring constantly, until mixture comes to a boil.

Reduce heat to low and continue to cook and stir until mixture thickens. Remove from heat. Pudding will continue to thicken as it cools. Allow to cool five minutes, then chill in refrigerator until completely cooled.

HOMEMADE MARSHMALLOWS

Serves 6 – 8

4 pkgs unflavored gelatin	2 C sugar
1 C cold water	2 egg whites
2 C GF powdered sugar, sifted	parchment paper

Line a cookie sheet with sides with parchment paper. Heavily coat with sifted powdered sugar, covering paper completely.

In medium saucepan soak the gelatin in cold water, stirring until soft. Add sugar and gently dissolve over low heat, about 5 minutes. Remove from heat and allow to cool until next step is completed.
In large bowl beat egg whites until stiff peaks form and then fold in the powdered sugar. While mixer is on low, slowly pour in the cooled gelatin mixture. Increase speed and beat until white and thick. Mixture should double in size.

Pour marshmallow mixture onto lined cookie sheet. Dust with more sifted powdered sugar, covering completely. Leave out overnight or for at least 3 hours to set. Marshmallows should be light and springy when set.

Move slab of marshmallows on parchment paper to counter. Using a large knife, slice marshmallows into 2" squares. This is best accomplished by sliding tip of knife through marshmallows from one end of the parchment paper to the other, rather than cutting in a sawing motion. Peel marshmallow squares off parchment paper. Store in airtight container or zip lock bags.

BOILED FROSTING

Frosts one cake

1 ½ C granulated sugar
¼ tsp GF cream of tartar
2/3 C boiling water
2 egg whites
1 tsp GF vanilla

In large, heavy saucepan mix sugar with cream of tartar. Add boiling water, stirring until sugar is dissolved.

Bring mixture to a boil over medium heat. Boil rapidly, without stirring, for 10 minutes until mixture reaches soft ball stage.

Remove mixture from heat and set aside while you beat the egg whites.

In large bowl beat egg whites until stiff. Slowly pour a thin stream of syrup into egg whites, beating constantly with electric mixer. Continue to beat frosting until frosting has cooled to warm and is of spreading consistency. Stir in vanilla.

Frost cake immediately, or refrigerate frosting until ready to use.

DEVILED EGGS

Serves 6

6 hardboiled eggs
½ C GF mayonnaise
2 Tbl finely chopped onion
1 tsp Lawry's seasoned salt
½ tsp salt
¼ tsp pepper
½ tsp GF dried basil
GF paprika

Cut eggs in half lengthwise. Gently remove yolks, being careful not to break whites.

In medium bowl mash egg yolks with fork. Add onion and seasonings to egg yolks, stirring to combine. Add mayonnaise and stir until smooth.

Spoon egg yolk mixture into egg white halves. Sprinkle with paprika. Refrigerate until ready to eat.

GREEN EGGS & HAM

Serves 4

6 eggs
1 C cooked ham, cubed
¼ C soy milk
½ tsp Lawry's seasoned salt
Salt & pepper to taste
6 drops green GF food color
3 Tbl GFDF margarine

In large bowl combine eggs and soy milk until well blended. Stir in ham, food color, seasoned salt, salt and pepper.

Heat margarine in large skillet until melted. Pour egg mixture into pan. Cook over medium heat, stirring gently until all egg mixture is cooked through.

Serve immediately

GLUTEN-FREE, CASEIN-FREE MACARONI & CHEESE

Serves 4

2 C cooked GF elbow pasta
1 C vegan dairy-free cheese
¼ C soy milk
½ tsp Lawry's seasoned salt
½ tsp GF dried basil

Cook the pasta according to manufacturer's directions. Drain and set aside.

In large saucepan combine remaining ingredients. Cook on low heat until cheese melts, stirring constantly. Add pasta to saucepan and stir until thoroughly combined.

** The best brand of cheese for good mac and cheese is "Vegan Gourmet®" Dairy Alternative Cheddar – this actually MELTS!**

GLUTEN-FREE, CASEIN-FREE PIZZA

Makes 1 – 16" crust

1 C brown rice flour
1 C tapioca flour
1 C potato starch flour
1 ½ tsp xanthan gum
2 tsp granulated sugar
¾ tsp salt
2 pkgs dry yeast
1 – 1 ½ C water, divided
2 eggs, lightly beaten
2 Tbl vegetable oil
1 tsp apple cider vinegar

Preheat oven to 400 degrees. Grease two large pizza pans or cookie sheets. Sprinkle with cornmeal. In small bowl combine dry yeast with sugar and ½ C warm water. Set aside until top is foamy.

In large bowl combine dry ingredients. Add 1 C water, eggs, oil and vinegar. Add yeast mixture and beat for 5 minutes until dough is smooth but not runny, adding more water if necessary. Spoon dough onto prepared pans. Oil hands and press crust to edges of pans.

Prebake crust for 10 minutes. Remove from oven and top with sauce and desired ingredients. Return to oven and bake 15 – 20 minutes until cheese is melted and crust is brown.

NOTES TO PARENTS

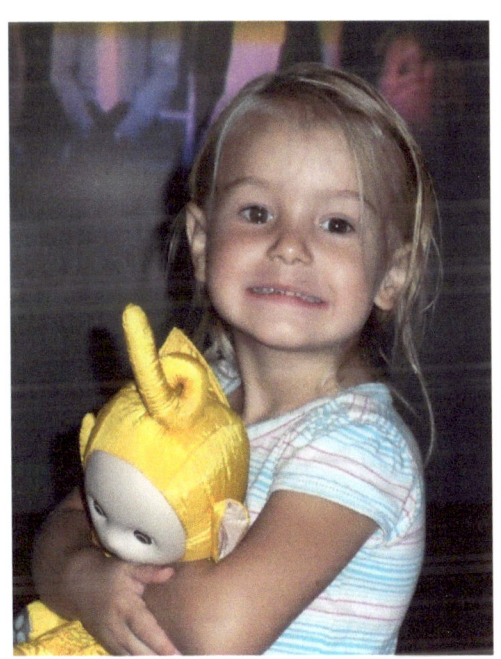

This book was written to help children who follow a gluten-free or a gluten-free & casein-free lifestyle explain to other children why they need to eat "special" foods. Morgan combined photos and a story in words that children can understand in order to teach children about gluten, casein, food allergies and cross-contamination.

Morgan's sister, Aivah, was diagnosed with Celiac disease and a casein allergy when she was 14 months old. She is now a happy, delightful 3 year old and follows a strict gluten-free and casein-free diet. She was one of the lucky ones who was diagnosed very young.

1 in 130 people have Celiac disease, an allergy, sensitivity or intolerance to gluten, although many have never been diagnosed. Celiac disease, gluten allergy and intolerance are very often misdiagnosed. Celiac disease, food allergy and food intolerance/sensitivity are not the same thing.

A food allergy is an immediate immune system response to a food you have eaten. An allergic response occurs within minutes, or up to an hour or so, after eating the food you are allergic to. You may experience itching or tingling in your mouth, stomach or abdominal cramps, skin rash or hives, diarrhea and/or vomiting. In severe cases, this may cause an asthmatic attack because the histamines your body produces have reached your lungs. A food allergy, such as an allergy to tree nuts or peanuts, may cause anaphylactic shock, a life-threatening reaction.

A food intolerance, on the other hand, is a delayed reaction to eating an offending food. The symptoms may be the same as those of a food allergy, but the delayed reaction can take hours or days to appear. A food intolerance is more difficult to diagnose, because of the delayed reaction, and can have long-term consequences.

When we eat food, our stomach creates gastric juices to digest the food we have just eaten. From the stomach, this mixture of food and gastric juices pass to the small intestine. Here, the pancreas and gallbladder help to break down the food into proteins, carbohydrates and fats. Our body is able to absorb these nutrients in the form of amino acids (proteins), monosaccharides (carbohydrates) and fatty acids (fats). The parts of the food that can't be broken down into amino acids, monosaccharides and fatty acids are passed onto the large intestine and are eliminated.

GLUTEN

The symptoms of Celiac disease, gluten allergy and gluten intolerance are very similar and result from the inability of the small intestine to absorb nutrients from food as it is digested. Celiac disease is an autoimmune disorder caused by the body's inability to digest gluten. Gluten is a protein found in grains such as wheat, rye and barley.

The inside of the small intestines is lined with small, finger-like projections called "villi". The villi absorb nutrients as the food passes through and pass the nutrients into our bloodstream. Gluten causes damage by irritating, flattening and shortening the villi. Damaged villi cannot absorb nutrients, resulting in malabsorption of the nutrients and malnutrition. Basically, the food your child eats is going in one end and out the other without stopping to leave behind the necessary vitamins, minerals and calories for proper nutrition. The small intestine is where iron, folic acid, calcium and Vitamins K, A, D and E are absorbed.

Imagine a train with many cars filled with vitamins, mineral and calories. Instead of making its scheduled stops at every town along the track, it races quickly along without stopping, dumping its cargo at the end of the track. The towns in between are going hungry
and are not thriving. This damage to the small intestine can also cause gluten, toxins and incompletely digested food to leak through the intestine into other parts of the body.

When we eat food, we sometimes take in antigens. Antigens are foreign substances, such as bacteria or toxins. When we take in antigens, our immune system's regulatory T-cells (white blood cells) recognize these antigens and destroy them so they won't harm us. Sometimes, our immune system doesn't work properly because of infections, stress, medications or other reasons. This causes our T-cells to stop regulating properly.

With Celiac disease and gluten sensitivity, our digestive system is not able to break down the gluten into amino acids. Our body sees the gluten as an antigen and creates antibodies to destroy it. Our body is working hard to try to break down the gluten into amino acids, while the antibodies are fighting to destroy the gluten. This creates inflammation in your intestines, which in turn can cause the villi to become damaged and flattened and allows the gluten and antibodies to pass into your bloodstream. When antigens enter our bloodstream, our body produces antibodies to fight and destroy the antigens.

When someone with Celiac disease eats foods that contain gluten, their immune system sees the gluten as a foreign substance and the body actually attacks its own cells.

Some possible symptoms of undiagnosed Celiac disease and/or gluten sensitivity are:

Skin disorders:

Blistered rashes on stomach, buttocks, arms, legs, neck (The medical term for this is Dermatitis Herpetiformis – DH); hives; psoriasis; eczema

Neurological disorders:

Loss of muscle coordination; headaches; migraines; behavioral problems

Digestive disorders:

Liquid, foul-smelling diarrhea; vomiting (at times projectile vomiting); distended abdomen; abdominal cramping; heartburn; constipation; excessive burping; ulcers (in mouth, esophagus, stomach, upper intestine)

Skeletal disorders:

Painful, swollen joints; soft bones

Other possible symptoms:

Weight loss; lack of muscle definition; high fever; listlessness; fatigue; inability to sleep through the night; dark circles under the eyes; Anemia or iron deficiency; low height and weight gain; asthma; chronic infections; irritability; lack of enamel formation on teeth

Unfortunately, the above symptoms can also be caused by other illnesses and diseases. If your child has a number of the above symptoms for any length of time, please consult with their doctor.

If left untreated, Celiac disease and gluten intolerance can cause permanent damage to the small intestine. It can become life-threatening and can lead to or exist in conjunction with other conditions such as:

Central and peripheral nervous system disorders (such as Multiple Sclerosis)
Osteoporosis, Osteopenia and other bone diseases
Painful, swollen joints (such as Lupus, arthritis)
Lack of dental enamel formation
Delayed start in menstruation
ADD / ADHD type symptoms, behavioral problems
Internal hemorrhaging
Severe weight loss; Anemia
Chronic Fatigue Syndrome
Fibromyalgia
Asthma
Diabetes
Thyroid disease
IBS (Irritable Bowel Syndrome)

DAIRY

Milk is made up of water, protein (casein), carbohydrates (a milk sugar called lactose), minerals, fats and other substances. A casein allergy is not the same as lactose intolerance. A casein allergy refers to the body's allergic reaction to casein, a protein found in dairy products. Lactose intolerance refers to the body's inability to digest lactose, a sugar found in milk.

An allergy occurs when our bodies react to the proteins in cow's milk, casein and/or whey, as if they were a foreign substance. This allergic reaction can occur within seconds to hours. Casein can cause an allergic reaction that can range from mild to life threatening. Mild symptoms may be a rash, hives or eczema. Symptoms may also affect the digestive tract causing bloating, cramps and diarrhea or respiratory reactions causing wheezing, difficulty breathing or asthma-like symptoms.

Lactose intolerance occurs when the small intestine does not make enough of an enzyme called lactase. Your body needs lactase to break down lactose. When lactose moves through the large intestine without being properly digested, it can cause symptoms such as gas, bloating and diarrhea. Lactose intolerance may have the same symptoms as an allergy, but intolerance symptoms generally take hours to days to appear. Some people who are lactose intolerant can't digest any milk products. Some people can eat small amounts of dairy products, or processed dairy products such as cheese without any physical problems.

AUTISM

1 in every 100 children is diagnosed with Autism. Many parents with Autistic children have seen improvements with a gluten-free, casein-free (GFCF) lifestyle. Some children with autism or Asperger's Syndrome cannot properly digest gluten or casein.

Eating these proteins leads to high levels of protein by-products, called gluteomorphines , in some children with Autism. These by-products may then affect behavior like an opiate drug would, altering the child's behavior, perceptions, pain messages, confusion level and their responses to the world around them. If gluten is removed from their diet, this reduces the level of gluteomorphines, and their perception and behavior improve.

Gluten and casein can become highly addictive opiates to children with Autism. Many children with Autism may prefer to eat only foods that contain gluten or dairy and are actually addicted to these foods. Some parents fear if they remove all gluten and dairy foods, their child will starve. There will be an initial "withdrawal" reaction, but once they are no longer eating gluten and casein, they will be more willing to eat other foods. Plain meat, fresh fruits and vegetables are all gluten-free and casein-free. Many parents have reported improved behavior and interaction after starting their child on a gluten-free, casein-free diet.

CROSS-CONTAMINATION

Cross-contamination occurs when a gluten-free food comes in contact with a food or a surface than contains gluten. Cross-contamination is a very real problem for those who follow a gluten-free diet. There are steps you can take to avoid cross-contaminating the gluten-free food. Gluten is invisible to the naked eye, but can contaminate surfaces such as counters, cutting boards and utensils.

You also need to remember that even though a product is listed as gluten-free, it must also be manufactured in a gluten-free plant to be truly gluten-free. Many manufacturers make products with gluten-free and/or dairy-free ingredients, but also manufacture products that contain gluten or dairy in the same plant. If so, there is a risk of cross-contamination. To be truly gluten-free and dairy-free, a food must be manufactured in a separate area where there is no chance of cross-contamination. Many companies state on their labels that the food is manufactured in the same plant as gluten and/or dairy products. Unfortunately, not all companies do this. The best way to find out if a product contains dairy or gluten or is manufactured in a gluten-free or dairy-free facility is to call the manufacturer or ask. You may have to talk to a few people to get to the right department, but it is well worth the effort.

Food isn't the only thing to be concerned with. Products such as toothpaste, lotions, shampoos, band-aids and medicines can also contain dairy or gluten. Gluten products are used as thickeners. Dried milk and/or dairy solids are commonly found in hair and body products. READ INGREDIENTS before purchasing anything. Believe me, this becomes second nature. Each time you pick up a product, you automatically turn it to the ingredient list before you consider purchasing it.

Cross-contamination can be a very big problem when eating in restaurants. A restaurant may advertise that they offer gluten-free foods. However, if they cook their gluten-free foods alongside the gluten foods, you no longer have gluten-free food. It has been contaminated by the gluten foods. If a restaurant uses the same utensils on gluten-free foods and gluten foods, your food is no longer gluten-free. Many people understand that foods need to be prepared with gluten-free ingredients. Unfortunately, they don't always understand the cross-contamination issues of using separate pans, dishes, utensils and preparation areas.
Always check WHERE the restaurant is cooking their gluten-free foods, and if they use separate cutting boards, pans and utensils. If they don't, you may want to consider eating at home.

As always – it is up to those following the gluten-free, dairy-free diet to determine if a product is safe for them.

OTHER NAMES FOR GLUTEN

Gluten is a special type of protein that is found in many grains. Gluten helps make baked goods elastic, giving it that "chewy" texture. This is why you need to add xanthan gum or guar gum to baked goods made with gluten-free flours. Without one of these ingredients, your baked goods won't hold together.

Gluten can be found in many foods. Everyone recognizes "wheat flour" or "flour". This is by no means a complete list, but a list of the most commonly used names for gluten:

Alcohol
Artificial colors
Barley
Bleu cheese (some Bleu cheese is made with bread – check ingredients)
Bran
Caramel color
Couscous
Dextrimaltose
Dextrins
Durum Semolina
Edible starch
Einkorn
Food starch (except pure cornstarch)
Groats
Hydrolyzed wheat protein
Hydrolyzed wheat gluten
Hydrolyzed wheat starch
Hydroxypropyltrimonium
Kamut®
Malt (flavoring, extract, syrup)
Miso
Modified food starch
Maltodextrin
Maltos (malt sugar)
Oats (oats do not contain gluten, but are generally cross-contaminated in the fields or manufacturing plants)
Semolina
Soy sauce (Gluten-free soy sauce is available, but must state gluten-free on the label)
Smoke flavoring
Spelt
Starch

OTHER NAMES FOR GLUTEN (cont)

Tabbouleh
Teriyaki sauce
Texturized vegetable protein (Vegetable protein made from soy is available)
Triticum Aestirum
Triticale (a hybrid of wheat and rye)
Vegetable starch
Wheat starch
Wheat protein
Wheat germ

OTHER NAMES FOR DAIRY

Dairy can be found in many foods and has many names. If your child has a casein allergy or is lactose intolerant please avoid the following:

Whey
Milk solids
Ammonium
Acaeinate
Demineralized whey
Hydrolyzed whey
Lactic Acid
Lactoferrin
Magnesium caseinate
Rennet
Whey protein
Casein
Calcium caseinate
Ammonium caseinate
Hydrolyzed casein
Iron caseinate
Lactalbamin phosphate
Lactoglobulin phosphate
Opta
Sodium caseinate
Lactose
Delactosen whey
Hydrolyzed milk protein
Potassium caseinate

Zinc caseinate
Lactate

I would like to thank my Nana for helping me and inspiring me through the process of writing this book. You taught me it takes determination and a lot of work, but it's all worth it. I would like to thank Aivah for inspiring me to find a way to help her and other kids with Celiac disease and a casein allergy.

Morgan Paulsen

About the Author

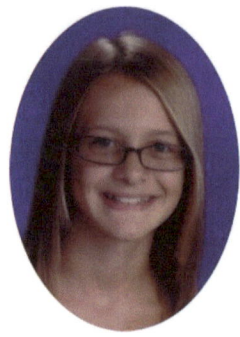

Morgan Paulsen is 12 years old and one of Aivah's older sisters. She is worried that when Aivah starts school, other children won't understand why she has to eat food that is "special". Morgan knows there are many young children who follow a gluten-free, casein-free lifestyle for various reasons. She wrote this book to help Aivah, and other children, teach their friends and classmates about the special foods they need to eat and the dangers of cross-contamination. Morgan's future plans are to become a Marine Biologist.

About the Photographer

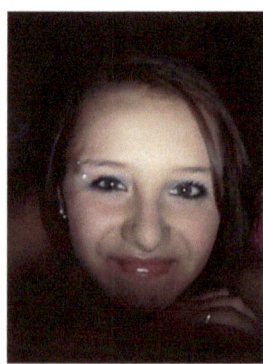

Emma Paulsen is 16 years old and Aivah's oldest sister. She loves photography and wanted to use her talents to help children visualize Morgan's story. Just like Morgan, Emma has been there through the worst of Aivah's reactions to gluten and casein. They have both held her and comforted her while she screamed for hours and have changed more nasty diapers than they care to remember. Both are pros at reading ingredient lists and are conscious of the dangers of cross-contamination. Emma is currently enrolled in an environmental science high school. Her college plans are to become a Forensic Pathologist.

About the Co-Author

Joyce Nielsen is the grandmother of Aivah, Morgan, Emma and 8 other grandchildren. She has over 30 years of experience researching and cooking for food allergies and special diets. She has experience with diets for Celiac disease, ADHD, Autism, Rheumatoid Arthritis, hyperactivity, lactose intolerance and casein allergy. She believes in a holistic approach to health that deals with the whole person rather than just treating symptoms. When Aivah was diagnosed with Celiac disease and a Casein allergy at 14 months of age, she created Don't Feed Me, LLC in an effort to share her knowledge of food allergies with others. Since its creation, Don't Feed Me, LLC has published a cookbook, "Don't Feed Me – Gluten-free, Dairy-free Cooking" and introduced a line of Allergy Alert T-shirts for children.

For more information about Celiac disease, food allergies and Sensitivities, cross-contamination and Autism visit our website at: www.dontfeedme.com

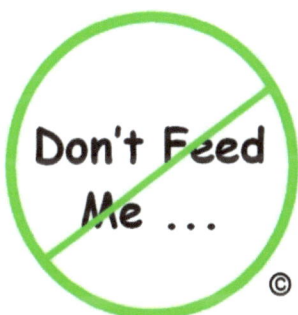

Send all questions and comments to:

joycen@dontfeedme.com

What Others Are Saying About This Book:

"The escalating number of children diagnosed with Celiac disease and similar food-related allergies should make us all more aware of how the most common ingredients can cause uncommon . . . and unnecessary effects. The child featured in this book went through an incredible transformation health-wise when her family learned the basics for treating her condition. Morgan Paulsen, her older sister, documents Aivah's path in a kid-friendly story with simple, fun recipes, and important notes for parents. It is a guide for children to understand and be compassionate of differences, and should cue all parents to reassess what their own children are eating."

Beatirice LaMonica
Writer and Home Health Advisor

"This book gives children the information they need to discuss gluten-free, casein-free eating with others. The easy-to-understand, personal nature of the book, in addition to the practical recipes, make it a must-have for anyone who is affected or knows someone who is affected by Celiac disease."

Janice Meintsma
Owner/President of Artistic Framing & Stained Glass

"Celiac Disease if affecting more and more families in the recent years and means a lot of lifestyle changes for kids and families alike. Aivah's book is a wonderful resource for kids who have been diagnosed with celiac disease and for their families. Especially with a new diagnosis, it is often helpful to know you are not going through this alone. The recipes in the back of the book are also a wonderful resource of tried and tested menus so you can ensure your child will be able to enjoy several of their favorite foods without feeling ill or having some of the uncomfortable symptoms associated with Celiac."

Dr. Amanda Leino, M.D.
Family Practice, Glencoe, MN

"I am very proud of both my girls for working together on this book. They have been through the worst of this disease as Aivah's siblings. They've seen what happens when Aivah eats the wrong foods and how happy Aivah is when she gets the foods she needs to stay healthy. They've both had to teach their friends what to do, and what not to do, when it comes to a cute little girl wanting to share their treats. Morgan and Emma wanted to find a way to help Aivah's friends understand this disease when she is old enough to start school and I feel they did an excellent job with the story, as well as the pictures. They both have big dreams for their futures and, as their mom, I feel that they have the potential to achieve every dream they have...and so much more. I love you girls!"

Mom
Angelica Jenneke